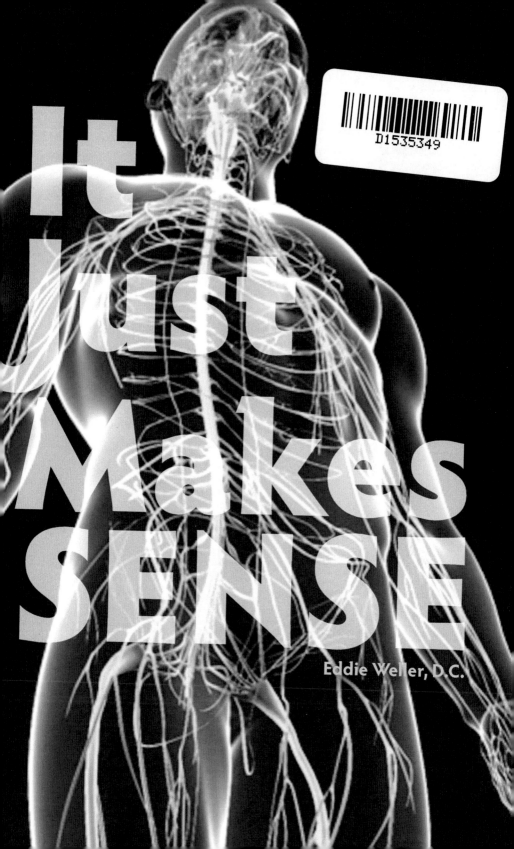

It just Makes SENSE

Eddie Weller, D.C.

IF YOU DON'T TAKE CARE
OF YOUR FAMILY, WHO WILL?

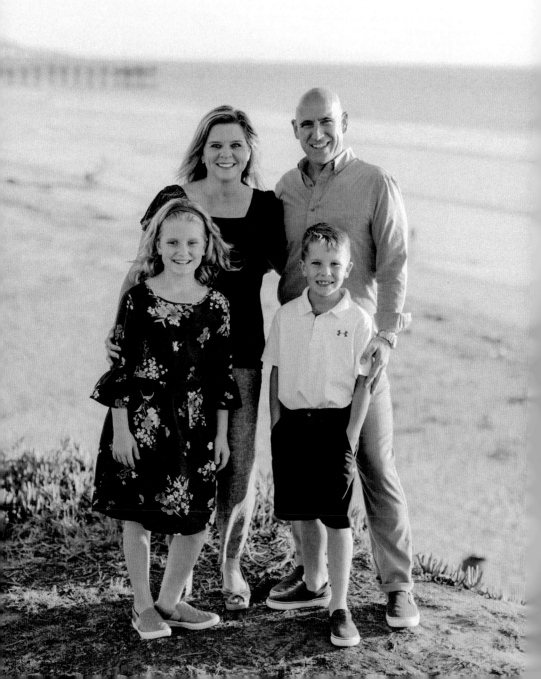

ABOUT THE AUTHOR
Eddie Weller, D.C.

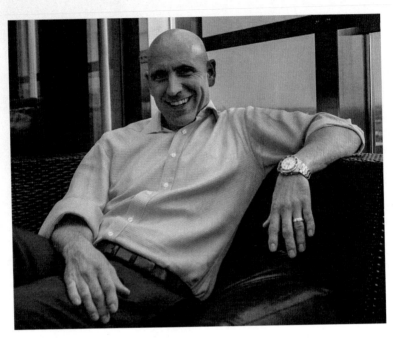

I have always had the desire to add to people's lives by giving them hope regardless of their situation. What most do not know about me is that I suffered with irritable bowel syndrome beginning at 17 years old. After graduating from high school, I moved to Florida to become a police officer. While in college and running a yacht detailing business, I was introduced to a man that would forever change my life. This man was a doctor who taught me about attaining health naturally and how the irritable bowel condition I was suffering from was related to my spine, particularly my nerve system. Very few know this about me either, but growing up, I struggled with reading comprehension. Irritable bowel and reading comprehension were no longer issues after having my nerve system restored via Upper Cervical Chiropractic, compelling me to become a Chiropractor. After graduating from Logan College of Chiropractic in 1998, I spent several additional years studying Upper Cervical Chiropractic because the Chiropractic school I attended did not teach the type of care that I now offer.

My life was transformed on so many levels that it became a struggle to come up with a fee for my care because, deep down, I knew it was priceless. My first Upper Cervical Chiropractic practice was unlike any other, operating completely on a donation basis for 3 years; it was my way of giving back. 10 years and 6 practices later, my heart led me to St. Louis after meeting my now wife. Just a short time after getting married, I opened a new office, where I was honored and fortunate to take care of people with conditions ranging from autism to allergies, colic to cancer, and depression to diabetes. I believe that regardless of the health issue, if the body has the opportunity to be neurologically sound, it then has the opportunity to build itself well again.

I currently own and operate "Getting Weller," host seminars and masterminds, as well as produce podcasts and online video courses ("TIC for the TOR") designed to train doctors in this unique form of Chiropractic. I have been honored to be the guest and keynote speaker on several TV shows, radio shows, and corporate events, as well as host my own commercials, infomercials, and a radio talk show.

I am blessed to have taught hundreds of students and doctors alike over the past 20 years and I will continue to mentor those seeking to learn how to deliver the Chiropractic message and upper cervical adjustment to the world.

People frequently state, "I want your energy." I am just trying to be the best version of me with a little bit of passion and excitement for what I do. Churches, schools, and work places frequently invite me to speak about how we all have the inborn potential to thrive and to live with purpose. I believe that most of us take yesterday's pain and bring it into tomorrow's pleasure, thus causing us to live a life of not enough. Well, not on my watch!

My motto is simple… If life is not fun, then what's the point of living it? I hope and pray that this book opens the door, answers a prayer, or simply gives you hope. A proper functioning nerve system helped me to live my "why" and it may just do the same for you.

To me, it just makes sense.

Eddie Weller, D.C.
Upper Cervical ChiropracTOR.

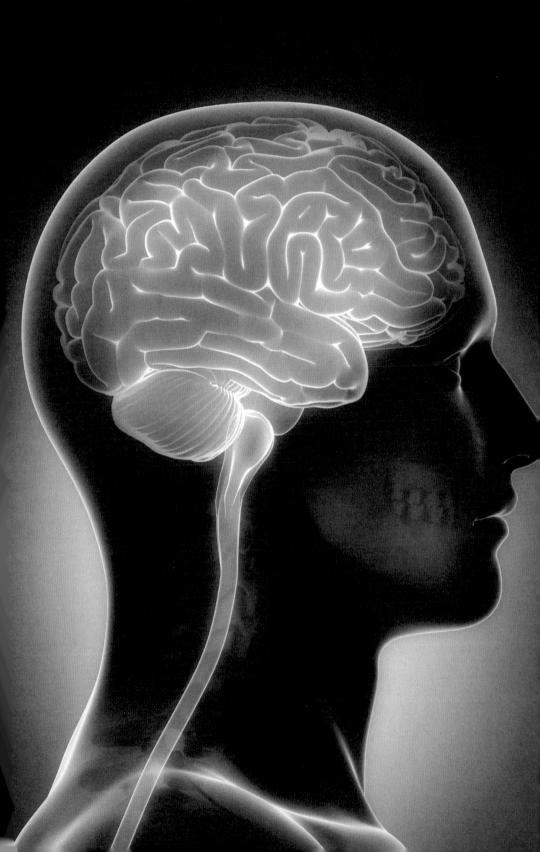

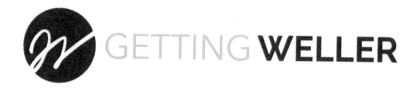

OUR MISSION:

WE HONOR AND SERVE THE BODY'S INBORN INTELLIGENCE BY ENSURING THAT YOUR NERVE SYSTEM IS FUNCTIONING PROPERLY THROUGH THE UPPER CERVICAL CHIROPRACTIC ADJUSTMENT. DOING SO ENSURES THAT YOUR BODY IS FUNCTIONING AT ITS OPTIMUM, ALLOWING THOUGHTS TO BECOME CLEAR AND LIFE TO BE EXPERIENCED AS IS WAS INTENDED TO BE... FULL OF HEALTH, ABUNDANCE, AND PURPOSE.

INTRODUCTION:
GROUND RULES

When playing baseball, the umpire typically goes over the ground rules to ensure that everybody from both teams (the coaches and players or, in this case, doctor and client) are on the same page. By doing so, the expectations are clear. The same rules apply here. Being "on the same page" is imperative when receiving this unique type of care.

There are several terms that are mentioned in this book that need to be defined and clarified before we get started. According to Merriam-Webster's Collegiate Dictionary (10th edition), the definitions for the terms "patient" and "client" are as follows:

Patient: an individual awaiting or under medical care and treatment

Client: one that receives a professional service from another

Medical patients are individuals who are typically treated for a short period of time with the intent to alleviate a symptom, sickness or ailment with the use of drugs or surgery.

By definition, "treatment" is an application of remedies given to a patient for a disease or injury; medicinal or surgical management; therapy. Therefore, treatment is what you receive from a medical practitioner.

Chiropractic: Chiro (hand) - Practic (adjustment)
Chiropractic is applying an adjustment to the spine done by hand. Nothing more and nothing less.

Subluxation: a condition in which the top two vertebrae in your spine misalign, causing the spine to be both neurologically and structurally compromised.

Adjustment: is a constructive, gentle force placed upon the subluxated (misaligned) vertebrae with the intent to restore structural and neurological function.

What We Believe...

There is that "extra-something" inside each and every one of us that gives us life. This spark of life that initially resided in a single cell had the divine blueprint of what makes you who you are today. This inborn "Innate" intelligence knows what to do and how to do it. The intelligence (that came from our creator) travels in and through your nerve system, which is commonly referred to as the neurological system. NEURO - LOGIC or intelligence within the nerve.

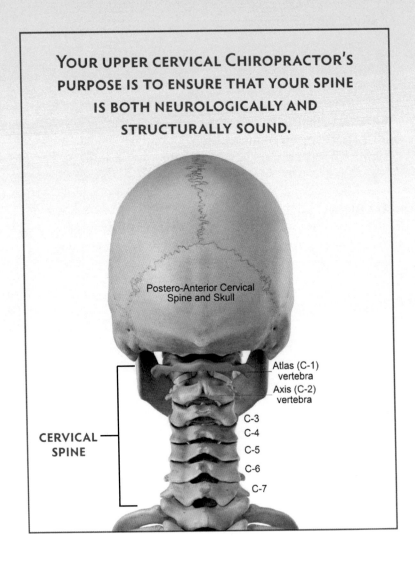

YOUR UPPER CERVICAL CHIROPRACTOR'S PURPOSE IS TO ENSURE THAT YOUR SPINE IS BOTH NEUROLOGICALLY AND STRUCTURALLY SOUND.

Postero-Anterior Cervical Spine and Skull

Atlas (C-1) vertebra

Axis (C-2) vertebra

C-3
C-4
C-5
C-6
C-7

CERVICAL SPINE

Every organ in the body, even the brain, needs proper nerve system function. Believe it or not, your brain does not keep you alive, but rather it is your brainstem. If you were to look up brainstem function, you would see that it controls your heart, lungs, digestion, and all of the countless involuntary functions that were divinely created to keep you alive.

The neurologic communication between the brain and the body through the brainstem is imperative for allowing the body the best ability to function at its optimum. We believe that the body does not need any assistance, just no interference to its functioning. As Upper Cervical Chiropractors, we focus on the uppermost portion of the spine because it protects the brainstem.

Having your spine checked for proper function, adjusted when needed and maintained your entire life, creates an opportunity to be the best version of you physically, psychologically, and spiritually.

MEDICINE BELIEVES THAT WE ARE SICK BECAUSE WE HAVE CANCER, DIABETES, HIGH BLOOD PRESSURE, ETC.

CHIROPRACTIC BELIEVES THAT WHEN WE HAVE CANCER, DIABETES, HIGH BLOOD PRESSURE, ETC. IT IS BECAUSE WE ARE SICK.

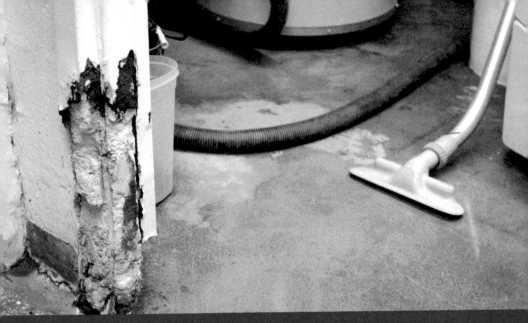

In other words…

Medicine focuses on removing the water in the basement (the effect)
Chiropractic seeks to find the hole in the roof (the cause)

Both professions have intentions to fix the house, they just simply have two different approaches.

This is why it is impossible for Chiropractic to be an alternative to Medicine or vice versa per the differences in both the approach and beliefs.

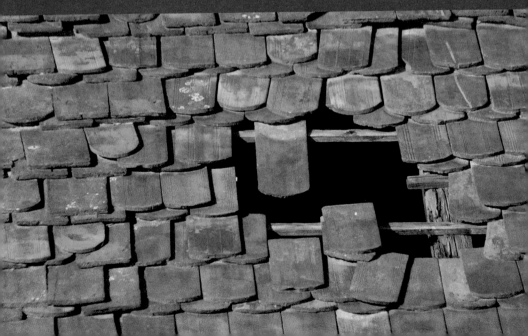

How It Works...

Step 1: Establish if the spine is neurologically compromised.

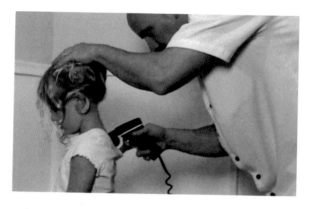

Step 2: Identify how the spine is "out of balance" (structurally compromised) with a postural analysis and spinal imaging via x-ray or CT.

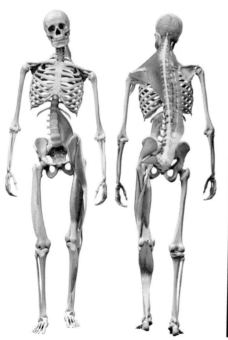

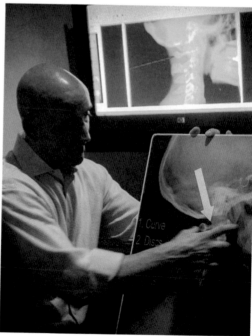

Table of
Contents

CHAPTER 1:

WHAT IS UPPER CERVICAL CHIROPRACTIC?

Your spine is separated into three parts: **CERVICAL, THORACIC,** and **LUMBAR.** The lumbar spine is your low back, the thoracic spine is the middle of your back (between your shoulder blades), and the cervical spine is what makes up your neck.

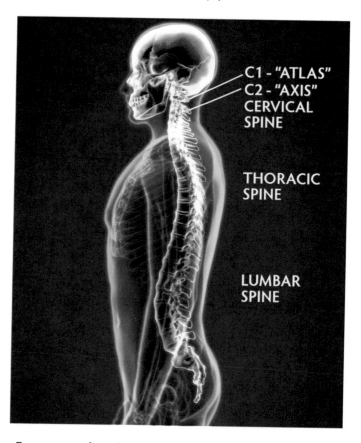

C1 - "ATLAS"
C2 - "AXIS"
CERVICAL
SPINE

THORACIC
SPINE

LUMBAR
SPINE

From your low back up towards your head, every vertebra stacks on top of one another and gets smaller in size, similar to building blocks. As elementary as it may seem, it gets quite complex when you get to the top of the spine. The top two vertebrae (C1 & C2, the upper cervical spine), also called the "Atlas" and "Axis," are unique compared to the other 22 vertebrae below. These two bones have their own distinct shape and a very important function, which is to support your head and to protect the most vital area in your body: the brainstem.

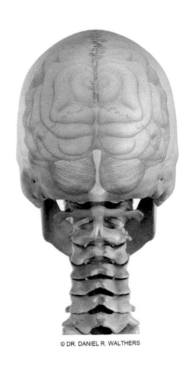

The upper cervical spine (particularly the C1/Atlas vertebra), is far more dynamic compared to the other 23 spinal vertebrae. The Atlas (C1) is the only bone in the spine that is held in place just by muscles, whereas the others feature a locking joint.

When you rotate your body or bend over to touch your toes, the locking joints within your spine limit movement because a nerve that gives the body life exits between each of the vertebrae / joints, and mobility beyond a certain range could potentially damage the nerve.

The fact that the Atlas is lacking an interlocking joint is a double-edged sword. It has far more mobility (notice how much more you can rotate your head in the "no" motion compared to how far you can rotate your lower body), but the tradeoff is less stability. When you experience a fall, bump your head, get in a car or sporting accident, or have emotional distress, the muscles are often unable to hold both the head and Atlas in place, causing the spine to become structurally compromised.

 UPPER CERVICAL CARE IS A STRICT DISCIPLINE OF CHIROPRACTIC THAT FOCUSES ON THIS VITAL AREA OF THE SPINE TO ENSURE THAT IT IS STRUCTURALLY AND NEUROLOGICALLY SOUND.

The Atlas vertebra supports the weight of the skull and it also protects the brainstem, the hub of your nerve system and the equivalent to the main electrical supply in your home. The brainstem is located at the base of the skull where the brain and spinal cord meet. Unfortunately, the same traumas that structurally compromise the spine also cause dysfunction within the nerve system. As Chiropractors, we call this condition a vertebral **SUBLUXATION**.

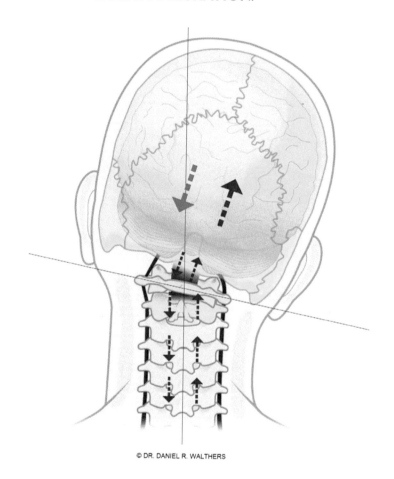

© DR. DANIEL R. WALTHERS

SUBLUXATION IS WHEN THE TOP TWO VERTEBRAE IN THE SPINE SHIFT OUT OF THEIR NORMAL POSITIONS CAUSING THE SPINE TO BECOME STRUCTURALLY AND NEUROLOGICALLY COMPROMISED.

CHAPTER 2:

THE HISTORY OF UPPER CERVICAL CHIROPRACTIC

Chiropractic was born on September 18, 1895. D.D. Palmer placed his hands onto a deaf man's spine and adjusted the second cervical vertebra (C2 / Axis) in his neck; the man's hearing was restored! A few years later, Palmer's son, B.J., took over Chiropractic and created hundreds of different ways to adjust the spine.

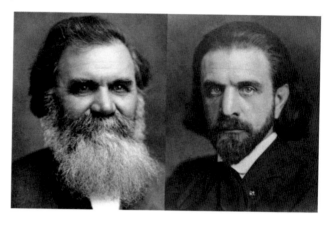

D.D. PALMER   B.J. PALMER

However, B.J. Palmer struggled because Chiropractors did not have any way to objectively gauge nerve system function within the spine. 1923 was a year that would forever change Chiropractic due to Dr. Palmer introducing an instrument called the "Neurocalometer" to the profession. His intention was to prove that if a Chiropractor analyzed the spine, located a misaligned vertebra, and adjusted that vertebra, that the nerve system would be constructively affected. This new instrument fulfilled that purpose. Unfortunately, it created controversy amongst Chiropractors as they thought Dr. Palmer created the instrument for the money; while many used the instrument in practice, others opposed its use.

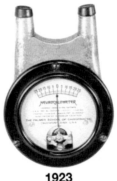

1923

"Neuro-Calo-Meter"

neuro = nerve / calo = heat / meter = gauge

As Dr. Palmer's research continued, his findings lead to greater focus on the upper cervical spine. In the spring of 1930, he introduced Upper Cervical Chiropractic to the profession. From that point on, all of his efforts, teachings, and research were based on the premise that the only place in the spine where you can affect the entire body neurologically, structurally (and psychologically) was the Atlas (C1) and Axis (C2) region (see Subluxation in Chapter 1) citing the anatomically unique features of this area of the spine.

During 16 years of Upper Cervical research (1935-1951), thousands of people were studied to prove the Upper Cervical theory. He had a staff of medical doctors performing medical exams while the only care that was provided was the adjustment of the Upper Cervical spine. The results were astounding and people traveled from all over the world to receive this type of care, including the wife of Dr. Charles Mayo, founder of the renowned Mayo Clinic.

Presently, there are 40 Chiropractic colleges worldwide with 100,000 graduated Chiropractors to date. However, there are just a handful of Chiropractic schools that teach the upper cervical method of analysis and adjusting.

CHAPTER 3:

FEELING TO FUNCTION

In order for a tissue cell to be healthy, it must be supplied with 3 essentials:

1.   Proper quantities of oxygen

2.   Proper quantities of nutrition

3.   Proper NERVE SIGNALS

Remember, a Subluxation is a condition in which the top two vertebrae in the spine become structurally compromised, causing a disruption of normal neurologic signals from the brain to the body.

There is only one place where the nerve system can become compromised and affect the entire body as a whole: the Atlas and Axis vertebrae. This structural compromise leads to partial closure (stenosis) of the foramen magnum (hole in the base of the skull where the brainstem resides) causing an imbalance neurologically, thus creating an incoordination within the body also known in Chiropractic as "Dis-ease".

Health is about FUNCTION

We frequently hear:

- "My neck is OK, but my hip is bothering me."

- "I don't have a spine problem; I have digestive issues."

- "What does my neck have to do with IBS, high blood pressure, or arthritis?"

- "How is this supposed to help me with a herniated disc in my low back?"

- "Why would I come see you if I don't have a neck problem?"

- "Why would a baby or child need to have their spine adjusted?"

The list of questions or comments is lengthy. As a client, you deserve to have your questions answered when it comes to your health and well-being. So let us go back to before you were even born.

Have you ever wondered about the first thing that was formed after conception? Was it your head? Lungs? Heart? Spine? Most never really give it any thought, as it just happens without us thinking about it.

Most would agree that there is a creator, a master controller or intelligence that makes life happen. Unfortunately, most also take their bodies for granted, especially when it comes to health. Well, in the divine moment that the sperm and egg united, a single cell was formed. That cell had 23 chromosomes from your mother and 23 from your father; and that cell did something beyond comprehension...it split. To this day, no scientist or doctor has yet to figure out exactly how. That single cell split and split and split and continued to do so until the notochord or neural streak was formed. The neural streak is from where your nerve system emanates.

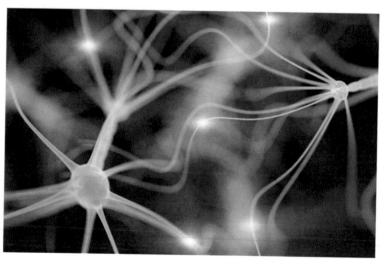

After the nerve system formed, the brain, heart, lungs, all of the other organs, bones, blood, arteries, veins, and every bit of your being followed. The trillions of cells that continued to multiply over a 9 month period were organized so perfectly that you were formed with eyes that could see, ears that could hear, a heart that pumped blood, feet for walking, and hands for touching, all of which occurred without any assistance from anyone or anything. We ALL were divinely created and were put here on Earth with intentional purpose.

It is through the nerve system that every tissue, organ, and cell is able to operate. The nerve system also plays a significant role in your emotional well-being; the brain is an organ similar to your heart, lungs, stomach, or liver, and it too depends on proper nerve system function. So, it is vitally important to ensure that your nerve system is functioning properly, thus giving you the best possible opportunity at life.

When focusing on symptoms or the removal thereof, why that symptom is present in the first place gets neglected. Symptoms are your body's way to communicate with you (like an alarm system), keeping you up to date on the status of how you are functioning. You can feel great and be healthy or you can feel terrible and be sick, but you can also feel great and be sick or feel terrible and be healthy.

 HEALTH SHOULD NEVER BE GAUGED ON HOW WELL ONE IS FEELING, BUT RATHER ON HOW WELL THE BODY IS FUNCTIONING.

When taking medication aimed at masking a symptom, your body is forced to work overtime as it attempts to resolve the underlying issue while also having to combat the synthetic substances within the medications. Pharmaceuticals are created to either speed up (stimulate) or slow down (inhibit) nerve function. In other words, the intention may be to help remove the condition, but the majority of the time, it is the symptom that gets targeted rather than the causative problem. Think about those that have had cancer and were "healed" who yet again get diagnosed and told that it "came back." That is because the core issue was never resolved or cured; it was just held at bay (remission) with the use of medications.

Please understand that medications can work for what they were created to do (i.e. treat symptoms). However, it is important for you to know that medicine is NOT intended to make you healthy, but just to treat disease or sickness. There are over 140,000 different types of diagnoses to describe what ails you and they all have one thing in common: an abnormally functioning nerve system.

> **WE MUST ALWAYS KEEP IN MIND THAT IF THE PROBLEM COMES FROM THE INSIDE, SO MUST THE SOLUTION TO THAT PROBLEM.**

When it comes to your health and well-being, your internal environment must be free of any obstructions or stressors. The subluxation obstructs your nerve system's ability to function normally, and the adjustment is intended to restore proper function. Physical, Chemical, or Emotional stress (see Chapter 8) always impacts the body in a negative fashion because it affects the nerve system, too. Alleviating as much stress as possible creates a more ideal environment for the spine to begin to "hold" the adjustment for a prolonged period of time; a key component of regaining and maintaining health, thus shifting from DIS-EASE back to EASE.

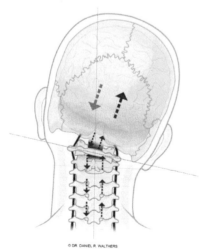

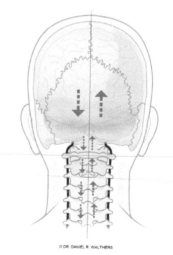

© DR. DANIEL R. WALTHERS

ABNORMAL NERVE FUNCTION
SPINE IN THE STATE OF
"DIS-EASE" "SUBLUXATED"

NORMAL NERVE FUNCTION
SPINE IN THE STATE OF "EASE"
(UN-SUBLUXATED)

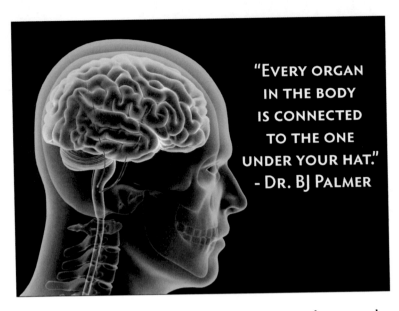

"EVERY ORGAN IN THE BODY IS CONNECTED TO THE ONE UNDER YOUR HAT." - DR. BJ PALMER

Always keep in mind that the entire spine adapts to the position of your head and that the positioning of your head is determined by the proper alignment (placement) of the Atlas vertebra. Once the Atlas (or Axis) vertebra is adjusted, the majority of the time, there is no reason to attempt to move other vertebrae within the rest of the spine because any of the misalignments below the Atlas vertebra are typically compensations due to the shifted position of the head. Similar to a snake, where the head moves, the body follows. Recall that, unlike your Atlas, the other spinal vertebrae have a locking joint to keep them in place, meaning they cannot misalign in the same manner as C1.

The goal and intention of Upper Cervical Chiropractors is to find and adjust the subluxation in order to ensure that your nerve system is functioning at its optimum. Care for each individual is very specific and "tailor-made," as no two misalignments (subluxations) are alike and, therefore, no two Upper Cervical Chiropractic adjustments are alike either.

REMEMBER, HEALTH SHOULD NEVER SOLELY BE BASED ON HOW WELL ONE IS FEELING, BUT RATHER ON HOW WELL ONE IS FUNCTIONING.

CHAPTER 4:

THE SCIENCE BEHIND UPPER CERVICAL CHIROPRACTIC

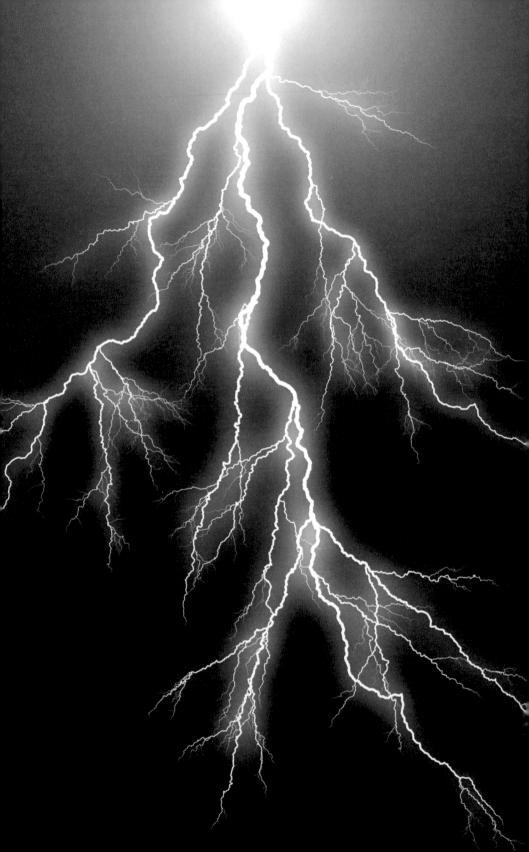

It has been said that we can survive without food for about 3 weeks, without water for about 3 days, and without air for about 3 minutes. However, without nerve function for a single second, life ends; because without nerve function, life as we know it would not exist. The human body and all of its organs are controlled by the nerve system.

WHEN A LIGHTNING BOLT HITS THE GROUND, IT USUALLY CREATES A FIRE. THAT IS BECAUSE WHEN THE PATH OF ELECTRICITY IS ALTERED, THE BY-PRODUCT IS HEAT.

The nerve signals from the brain to the body travel at just about 270mph. Just like lightning, these signals are electrical. When the Atlas vertebra is subluxated, it disrupts the normal electrical signals within spine, and in turn creates heat. Hence the importance of the invention of the neurocalometer (NCM) (see Chapter 2: History). However, since the inception of computers, today's Upper Cervical Chiropractor utilizes infrared thermography to gauge the function of the nerve system.

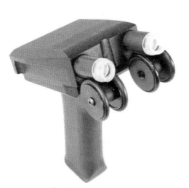

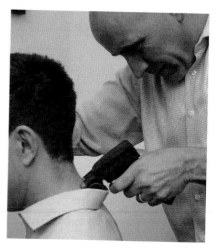

Infrared Thermography

Nerve signals travel from the brain and down the spinal cord, then exit the spine and connect to every organ, tissue, and cell of the body. One of those organs (the largest in the body) is your skin. Each of the nerves that exit the spinal column innervates (communicates and attaches to) specific areas of the skin, thus dividing the body into patterns known as "dermatomes."

The capillary beds (tissue just below skin) are always adapting to spinal (more specifically) nerve system function. Any irritation to the nerve system (primarily at the top of the spine) will cause the skin's natural temperature symmetry to fall out of balance; the elevated temperatures from one side to the other are indicative of interference to the electrical signals within the spine.

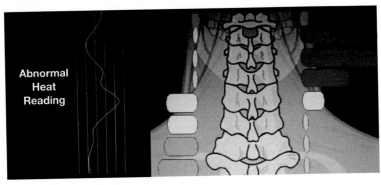

Abnormal
Heat
Reading

ABOVE ILLUSTRATIONS INDICATE A NEUROLOGICAL DISTURBANCE WITHIN THE SPINE.

Your upper cervical doctor utilizes infrared spinal thermography to identify if your nerve system is generating abnormal heat due to electrical (neurologic) dysfunction within the spine. Without the use of infrared thermography, your Upper Cervical Chiropractor would have no way of knowing if your spine is functioning the right or wrong way.

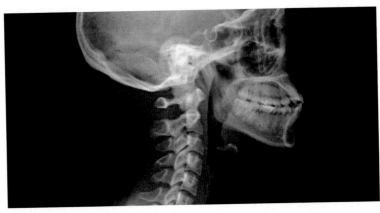

Then, x-ray or CT imaging is utilized to pinpoint the misalignment of the Atlas and/or Axis down to the nearest millimeter and degree, thus locating where the spine is being structurally compromised.

A gentle and specific adjustment returns the vertebra back into its normal position and, in turn, restores the body back to normal neurological function, as confirmed by the post-adjustment infrared spinal scan to ensure that the temperature asymmetry has been eliminated (see Chapter 11: Frequently Asked Questions).

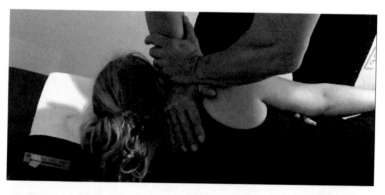

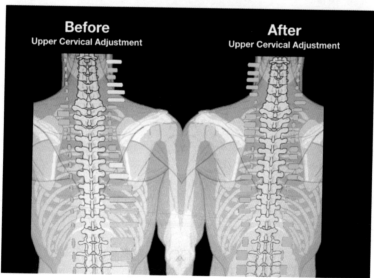

ILLUSTRATION OF BEFORE AND AFTER ADJUSTMENT. NOTICE THE DIFFERENCE IN TEMPERATURES FROM SIDE TO SIDE.

CHAPTER 5:

THE PROCESS OF UPPER CERVICAL CHIROPRACTIC CARE

The most important part of starting Upper Cervical Chiropractic Care is for your doctor to attain enough data to create a baseline of the current state of your spine; both structurally and neurologically. This requires several different types of exams that are performed throughout your first 3 visits. The day 1, 2, and 3 protocols are to ensure that your doctor attains enough neurologic data via infrared thermography to establish what is called your "pattern" reading.

DAY 1 (30-45 minutes):

You and your doctor will discuss your concerns and review your initial paperwork. Your doctor will then explain why many different tests and exams are required prior to starting care. Functional and structural evaluations will follow, and you will receive your 1st neurological examination. Once the data is collected, you will either be escorted to the X-Ray / CT imaging room, or in some cases, your doctor may refer you for imaging at an offsite location.

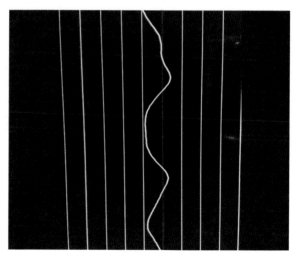

DAY 1 SCAN

DAY 2 (30 minutes):

Prior to your arrival, your doctor will have studied and reviewed all of the data collected from your day one exams. It is highly recommended that you bring your spouse, a family member, or a friend with you as the information covered can be a bit much to remember. You will learn the current state of your spine and how it correlates with your infrared spinal scan. Your doctor will then explain their findings and how it is affecting your health and well-being. Also during this visit, a second infrared spinal scan is performed and compared to your day one scan for similarity.

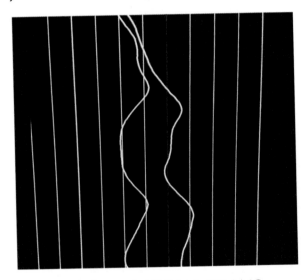

DAYS 1 & 2 SPINAL SCANS

The second scan is essential for your doctor to begin to establish your **abnormal neurologic baseline.** Lastly, you will be given your initial care program recommendations and will be prepared for your initial Upper Cervical Chiropractic adjustment, which is performed on day 3.

DAY 3 (45 - 60 minutes):

During your first two visits, your doctor attained neurologic data via two infrared spinal scans. A third spinal scan is required in order to give your doctor conclusive confirmation of your abnormal neurologic baseline reading. Think of it like a finger print, or in this case, a "spinal print." As upper cervical doctors, we call this your "pattern." Once all three scans are compared to one another, your pattern is then established. From this day forward, every future scan that your doctor performs will be compared to it.

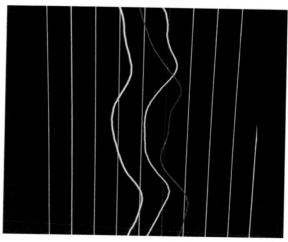

DAYS 1, 2 & 3 SPINAL SCANS

Before positioning you onto the adjustment table, your doctor will explain how the adjustment is performed. Once you are both on the same page, your doctor will then instruct you on how to position yourself onto the adjustment table. Prior to your first Upper Cervical adjustment, it is advisable that you use the restroom (or at least try) because getting up before the required resting time period is over may interfere with the setting of either the atlas or axis vertebra.

The majority of the Upper Cervical doctors will position both your head and body in a neutral position, as the adjustment itself requires very little force in order to move the vertebra out of its abnormal positioning, thus making the Upper Cervical adjustment safe for you and your loved ones of any age.

Once the adjustment has been performed, your doctor or a staff member will assist in sitting and standing you upright. It is imperative that you DO NOT get up on your own, as doing so will engage muscle movement prematurely and possibly cause your spine to return back to its abnormal position before the adjustment has fully taken hold. You will be escorted to a private resting suite, your head placed onto a contour pillow to support your spine, with pillows placed under your knees for lower body support; you will then be covered with a blanket. The purpose of the resting period is to give the muscles, ligaments, and joints ample time to adapt to the spine's new positioning. Absolutely no cellular phones are allowed in the resting suites as they will disturb others and will also keep you from relaxing properly.

After resting for up to an hour (future adjustments will require a minimum rest period of 30 minutes), you will be escorted back to the adjusting/scanning room and a post-adjustment spinal scan will be performed to ensure that your spine accepted the adjustment, as indicated by having your heat pattern no longer present. This will confirm that your nerve system has been restored to proper functioning.

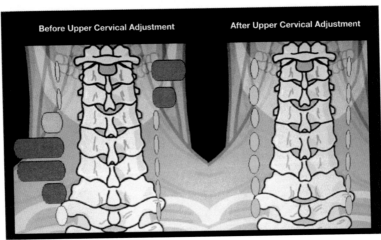

A follow-up visit will be scheduled within a week to identify if your spine is holding the adjustment.

RECAP OF DAYS 1, 2, & 3

DAY 1:

- One-on-one doctor consultation involving both a health and lifestyle assessment
- 1st infrared spinal exam
- Functional and Structural exams
- Attain spinal imaging (x-ray or CT)

DAY 2:

- Doctor consultation to review and explain Day 1 exam data
- 2nd infrared spinal exam
- Doctors recommendations for initial care plan
- Instructions in preparation for upper cervical spinal adjustment on Day 3

DAY 3:

- Payment made towards initial care program
- 3rd infrared spinal exam performed to confirm your baseline "pattern" reading
- Upper cervical adjustment performed followed by a 30-60 minute resting period
- Follow-up infrared spinal exam performed after resting period confirming the upper cervical adjustment was performed correctly

CHAPTER 6:

THE 2-4-6 RULE

The concept behind Upper Cervical Chiropractic Care is to ensure that your nerve system is functioning free of any compromise. Therefore, it is imperative for your doctor to collect accurate neurological data at each visit. To do so, we ask that you please follow the **2-4-6 Rule**.

- **2 hours** prior to your visit, NO NICOTINE or CHEWING GUM of any type

- **4 hours** prior to your visit, NO CAFFEINE or ARTIFICIAL SUGAR INTAKE

- **6 hours** prior to your visit, REFRAIN FROM TAKING ANY MEDICATIONS*

Besides what is stated above, there are other causes that can adversely affect your infrared spinal exam readings:

- Sweating from a hot day or from working out

- Damp hair from a shower

- Heat or air conditioning while in the car, directed towards the face

Failing to adhere to the 2-4-6 Rule or to eliminate the environmental factors will create inaccurate data and may create two separate consequences:

YOU MAY RECEIVE A SPINAL ADJUSTMENT
WHEN IT WAS NOT NEEDED

OR

YOU MAY NOT RECEIVE A SPINAL ADJUSTMENT
WHEN IT WAS NEEDED

Although medicine will alter your healing ability, your Upper Cervical Doctor does not prescribe or take you off of any types of medication. In the event that you decide to get off of your medication(s), that decision is between you and the prescribing doctor. In regards to nicotine and artificial sugars, it is recommended that you stop using them all together.

CHAPTER 7:

EXPECTATIONS

Many people that are introduced to Upper Cervical Chiropractic have experienced other types of Chiropractic, as well as other modalities such as physical therapy, occupational therapy, medication and/or surgery, unfortunately, often attaining unsatisfactory results. When you are disappointed with either a health care or professional service provider, it is typically due to expectations not being met. Being on the same page helps set an expectation for both you and your doctor in order for you to receive all of what Upper Cervical Care can provide.

WHAT TO EXPECT

- Timely appointments

- Neurological spinal exams on every visit

- Your doctor to adhere to the Day, 1, 2 & 3 protocols

- Invitations to appreciation and educational events

- Your information to be held confidential and secure

- A peaceful and nurturing environment

In today's world, there are many doctors who treat you like a number instead of taking care of you as if you were a family member. If at any time you find yourself unsure or in need of assistance regarding an issue or question, please know that your concerns are a top priority. Upper Cervical Chiropractors strive to provide the best possible care to ensure that both you and your family have a pleasant experience. A mind at peace, along with having confidence in your Doctor, is the cornerstone of giving your body the best ability to heal.

WHAT NOT TO EXPECT

Your Upper Cervical Chiropractor strives to be upfront and transparent when it comes to this unique type of care. Unfortunately, depending on state laws, Chiropractors perform many different services that are either unnecessary or unrelated to Upper Cervical Care. When receiving Upper Cervical Care, you will not have...

- Your spine twisted, pulled, "cracked" or "popped"

- Massage

- Acupuncture

- Physical therapy (ice, heat, muscle stimulation, ultrasound, etc.)

- Low back, arm, or leg manipulations

- Your spine adjusted on every visit (as our goal is for you to hold the adjustment for a prolonged period of time)

- Your Upper Cervical Chiropractor take you off of medications (that is between you and your prescribing doctor)

- Your health issue to be resolved immediately. All health processes, good and bad, take time; it takes time for your body to build itself sick or well.

We do not aim to replace any other type of care that you may be receiving. The principles and practices regarding Upper Cervical Chiropractic are not about treating a disease or resolving a diagnosed condition, but rather creating a healthy neurological environment to enable your body to function at its optimum. By doing so, thoughts become clearer, and your body is then able to adapt to life's every day stressors much easier.

CHAPTER 8:

THE "3-Ts"

Believe it or not, one of the most important tasks your nerve system has is to adapt to life's daily stressors. In the Chiropractic world, we call these stressors the "3-Ts." The influence of the following stressors can affect the body in many different ways...

THOUGHTS
TRAUMAS
TOXINS

1. **THOUGHTS** (emotions) cause the nerve system to either speed up or slow down depending on how your mind reacts to that stressor. Having a bad day, getting frustrated with traffic, arguing with someone, being aggravated/frustrated at work, having financial issues or relationship conflicts... let's be honest: WE ARE HUMAN! The truth is that stress of some sort will always be present. Heck, most have it daily. The point is: your nerve system is always "on the job," it is always responding and adapting to life's stressors. Depending on how long you hold onto what is causing the emotional stress (like taking yesterday's pain into tomorrow), these stressors can create many different types of health issues.

Some of them are...

- Digestive problems (ulcers and irritable bowel)

- Insomnia & Chronic fatigue

- Skin irritations and Rashes

- Thyroid complications

- Irregular heartbeat & High blood pressure

- Depression/Anxiety

2. Ever watch America's Funniest Home Videos? For some reason, we put ourselves in the strangest predicaments and the consequences are either slipping down the stairs or a cliff, getting hit in the head with an object, and/or a sporting injury. Most, however, never think about the common **TRAUMATIC** forces experienced such as birth, the process of crawling to walking, texting, watching TV in bed with the head propped

up, sleeping on your stomach, being rear ended while driving, poor ergonomic positions at work, improper form while exercising, etc. (the list goes on and on), all of which can shift the spine out of its normal position causing the nerve system to become compromised.

3. Your environment (either internal or external) plays a significant role when it comes to your health. For instance, medications, smoking, drinking too much alcohol, artificial sweeteners, the chemicals in food, etc. all produce a stress to the body. This stressor is known as a **TOXIN.**

You may ask yourself, "How do medications stress the body?" Well, have you ever watched or heard a drug ad on a TV or radio commercial, and once they state the drug's use, a quieter voice (along with happy people enjoying life) references all of the side effects?

IF SIDE EFFECTS INCLUDE HEADACHES, VOMITING, DIARRHEA, ORGAN FAILURE, SUICIDE OR DEATH, THEN THE MEDICINE MUST BE TOXIC."

There are also thousands of toxic chemicals, with exposure both voluntary and involuntary, in cleaning supplies, body soaps, lotions and deodorants, diet food products, and sugarless candy. Over time, these types of substances can stress the body enough to cause the immune system to work overtime as it seeks to fight off the toxins in an attempt to maintain your health.

To recap, when the body is unable to ward off a chemical, guard against a physical traumatic injury/incident, or protect itself from emotional stress, the result will eventually override the body's ability to adapt to one or many of these stressors, causing the spine to become subluxated. When the spine subluxates, normal / healthy nerve system function stops.

"IF WE LOOK DIFFERENT ON THE OUTSIDE, WE MUST ALSO LOOK DIFFERENT ON THE INSIDE."

As you may have noticed, the body is less capable of maintaining a healthy state or building itself well when the stress from thoughts, traumas, or toxins are present. Therefore, a person receiving Upper Cervical Chiropractic care should not expect to regain a normal state of health or function immediately, as it has taken years for your body to grow into the abnormal state it is in.

Mechanics tune up your car with the goal of having it operate / run to the best of its ability based on what they have to work with. Some cars are parked outside, while others are in a garage. Some run over potholes or get bumped in a parking lot, while others have had the motor blow out, transmission failure, or the airbags deployed.

Some people may have had a fall, a sports injury, the occasional fever, cold, or headache. Others have had cancer, surgery, extensive arthritis, bone degeneration, loss of normal spinal curves, etc., while others may show very little abnormal changes. Just like the mechanic, your Upper Cervical Chiropractor aims to "tune up" the body as they too are going to do the best they can with what they have to work with.

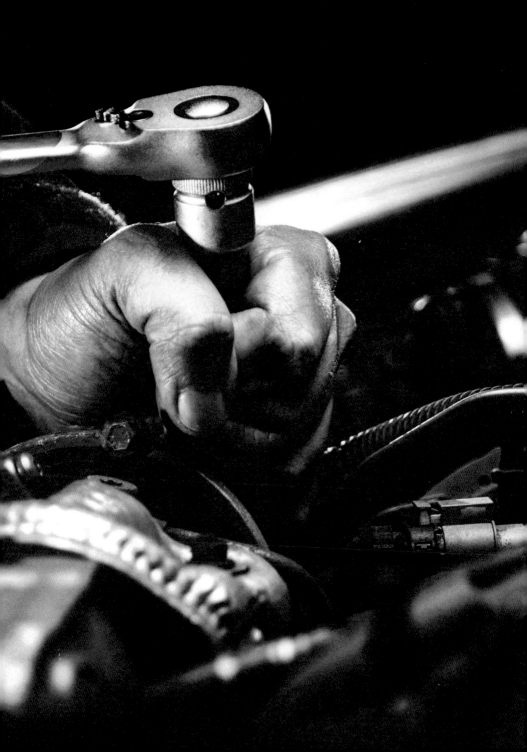

CHAPTER 9:

MAINTAINING (OR "HOLDING") YOUR ADJUSTMENT

Your nerve system controls everything that happens in your body, from digesting the food you ate today to pumping 2,000 gallons of blood from your heart, to even the fact that you can read and comprehend this text; it is a miracle, really. Such is why health should not be determined by how one is feeling, but rather by how well the body is neurologically functioning.

Holding, or maintaining, the adjustment means that your infrared thermographic / neurologic scans (and other exams) are indicating that your spine does not yet require another adjustment. Recovery time is directly proportional to how long your adjustments hold because, like eating right, exercising, or getting enough rest, it is the consistency of keeping your nerve system functioning properly that allows you to heal naturally. The concept behind Upper Cervical Care is to create a healthy neurological environment for your body; the power ("life source") that flows through the nerves is what gives the body life. When you maintain your adjustment longer and more consistently, the stronger your nerve system function will be and the greater the health benefits you will receive.

Your spine may only need a few adjustments during the initial phase of care, and that is a good thing! It is similar to watering a plant; it would be foolish to water the plant 2 to 3 times per week when the soil is still moist; over-watering the plant would create an unhealthy environment for it. The same is true when it comes to adjusting your spine. Less, in this case, is undoubtedly more, as the intention of Upper Cervical Doctors is to allow your body the opportunity to do the best that it can by facilitating your nerve system to function at its optimum. Just like watering the plant, your spine will be adjusted only when it needs it.

Neurologic spinal examinations will therefore be performed on every visit to determine if your spine is holding the adjustment or not.

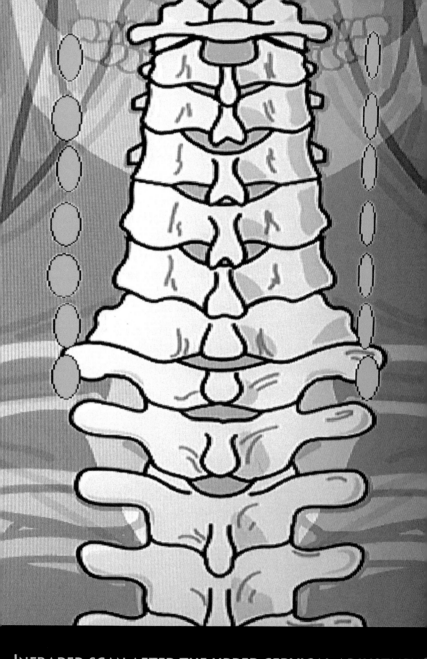

INFRARED SCAN AFTER THE UPPER CERVICAL ADJUSTMENT
"PATTERN" IS NO LONGER PRESENT

It is important to understand that the 3-Ts discussed in the previous chapter do not just cause the Atlas or Axis misalignment, but they are also the reasons why you lose your adjustment / no longer hold. To recap, the 3-Ts break down as follows:

EMOTIONAL STRESS (THOUGHTS)
PHYSICAL STRESS (TRAUMAS)
CHEMICAL STRESS (TOXINS)

By recognizing each one of these different stressors in your life, you will be able to assist your body in holding for a prolonged period of time. Emotional stressors are the number one trigger that will cause you to "go out" of adjustment. This type of stress can take months to years to resolve. More often than not, it is due to relationships; relationships with family or friends or co-workers all play a role in your spinal/neurological function.

Physical stressors such as birth trauma, falling out of a tree as a kid, sleeping on the wrong type of pillow, being on the computer all day, or scrolling through your smart phone apps for a prolonged period of time ("text neck") can cause your spine to be in a compromised position. These types of stressors create an environment that makes it difficult for your body to maintain or hold your Upper Cervical adjustment.

Chemical stressors are everywhere; in the food that we eat, the beverages we consume, the air that we breathe, the supplements and pharmaceuticals we take, etc. Your body is exposed to chemical stressors almost constantly.

It is no wonder why the world is so sick. Your body is dealing with so many different stressful environments that, sooner or later, the stressors overcome the body's ability to maintain itself.

Since these past and present stressors can inhibit your spine from holding an adjustment, your Upper Cervical Doctor may recommend that you work in conjunction with him or her and with a coach or counselor, dietician, and/or personal trainer or physical therapist.

Your primary goal should be to eliminate as many of the 3-Ts from your life that you can. When starting care, typically your doctor will want to see you once or twice per week for the first few weeks of care, then taper off to once every 1-2 weeks for the next few months. Most initial care programs are 12-16 weeks in length. Keep in mind, in most circumstances, you should not need to have your spine adjusted frequently (more than twice per month), but rather, only when your spine goes out of adjustment (becomes subluxated). The majority of the office visits will vary in length from 10-30 minutes depending on whether you get adjusted or not. The purpose of the visit frequency is to establish how long your spine holds the adjustment. It is when your spine is holding the adjustment that enables the body to shift from a degenerating state to a regenerating one.

An initial Upper Cervical Care plan is structured so that your doctor has enough data to establish how long your spine is holding the adjustment, and all of your future visits will be predicated on how well you hold. For instance, your doctor will probably want to space your visits out to 2-3 visits a month if you are holding for 2 weeks between adjustments. If you are holding for a longer period of time, your visit schedule will be case dependent based on your doctor's recommendations.

Once the initial care plan is completed, a maintenance care program will be created for you, as well as other additional recommendations aimed to help you attain the desired results. Some people may only hold their adjustments for a few weeks at a time while others may hold for several months. It is important to have your spine checked all the same. You change the oil in your car every three months, you visit the dentist every six months, you have a physical once a year; your spine is very dynamic, so it just makes sense to have it checked regularly.

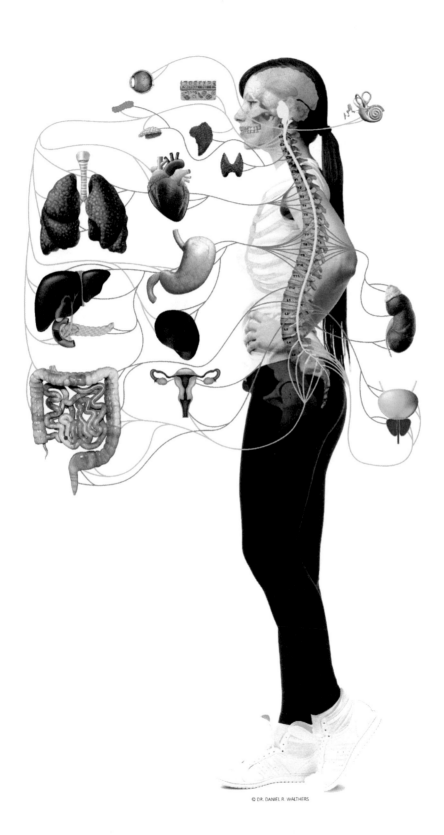

CHAPTER 10:

RETRACING

At the very moment your spine receives an Upper Cervical Chiropractic adjustment, everything changes; it is like turning up the dimmer switch to a light to give the bulb all the power it needs to be as bright as possible. Some people notice their sinuses and breathing immediately change while others may feel completely calm or full of energy. The reason why there are so many different types of reactions is because no two spines or nerve system compromises are alike.

The body must then undo years of breaking down and work extensively to heal, repair, and restore itself well again. This restorative phase of care is called "RETRACING," and it is a healing state likely to be accompanied by some pain and discomfort, as the body must "retrace" its steps back through the process of breaking down, to the best of its ability of course.

At some point, your health took a turn for the worse. From that day on, the body's normal functioning processes became disrupted and subsequently fell into a state of "Dis-Ease" because there became a lack of "Ease" within the nerve system (see Chapter 3). During this healing phase of care (typically the first 4 – 6 months of care, though it comes in many different forms and phases), clients often experience symptoms that have not been present for months or even years. Some of the common signs of retracing are neck and back pain, joint pain, strange bowel movements, and fatigue. When these healing symptoms arise, the first impression of them is often that you are becoming worse, but your health is like a ladder with the top being where you strive to be and the lower rungs being where you typically start the process of regaining optimal function; retracing involves climbing back up the rungs that you hit as your health declined and working your way through the underlying issues that developed along the way. Rest assured that retracing is normal; it goes to show that healing is not necessarily easy.

As you can probably imagine, the older you are, the slower the process can be and the more limited the healing capability will probably be due to the amount of degeneration one has. It is similar to bringing an older car to a mechanic; you would not realistically expect the car to be returned to you as if it was new again.

"SO, HOW LONG DOES IT TAKE TO GO THROUGH THE RETRACING PROCESS?"

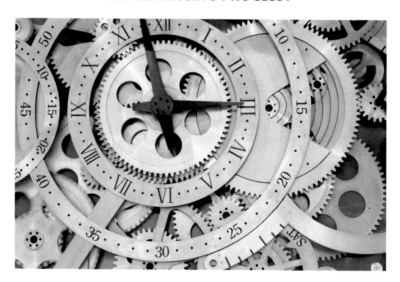

The question of time is a very sensitive subject because most of us do not like to experience any discomfort or pain during this healing / restoration process. Retracing is like working out; during the first few months of exercising, your body experiences pains that it has never experienced before because your muscles, joints, and ligaments are having to adapt to this new (although constructive) stress that it is experiencing. Trust that your body knows what to do and how to do it; when your nerve system is functioning properly, the body shifts from a degenerating state to a regenerating one. It is similar to weight loss; if it takes time to gain weight, then it must also take time to lose it.

CHAPTER 11:

FREQUENTLY ASKED QUESTIONS

"DO YOU ACCEPT MY INSURANCE FOR PAYMENT?"

If you were to Google "health insurance definition," it reads:

"Health insurance covers medical expenses for illnesses, injuries, and conditions."

Per the definition, insurance is based on treatments for a particular condition(s) that are deemed "medically necessary" over a period of time. The medical doctor's aim is to remove the symptom, usually with the use of medication or surgery. In order to do so, they must provide a "differential diagnosis" by creating four different possible diagnoses. Then, several tests are performed to rule out the three remaining diagnoses to hopefully treat you based on the correctly diagnosed condition, a key characteristic in the American "disease" or "sick care" system that has been labeled "healthcare." Of course, this forces people to allow their insurance carrier (not a doctor) to dictate the type of care you receive based on your condition's title (diagnosis).

Your insurance carrier and your primary doctor are unlikely to have been trained in Upper Cervical Chiropractic nor have they ever been educated about why you would need this type of care, especially if your Chiropractor is not treating any type of condition or disease. Upper Cervical Chiropractic is not about treating any type of medical condition, but rather geared towards restoring neurological function.

Consider the following scenario:

Your doctor performs a spinal scan, which reveals that your spine is holding the adjustment. This indicates that you would not require any type of care (adjustment) during that visit, similar to a dentist telling you that you do not have any cavities during a check-up. If your Upper Cervical Doctor were to bill the insurance company, a diagnosis code as well as a procedure code addressing the diagnosis must be provided. However, if your spine is found to be neurologically sound during that visit, there would be no way for your doctor to create a diagnosis. Therefore, if you do not need to be adjusted on that particular visit and your doctor chooses to bill the insurance anyway, that would be insurance fraud.

Insurance companies dictate when, where, and how much care one should receive, but your care should be between you and your doctor rather than a third party.

The purpose and intention of Upper Cervical Chiropractic is to ensure that your nerve system is functioning properly. When your spine is holding the adjustment, obviously you would not require any type of care or adjustment on that particular visit (recalling the old adage, "If it isn't broken, don't fix it"). Insurance companies do not recognize this type of protocol/care and they do not pay for the spinal scan or the analysis of the scan. According to most insurance providers, a Chiropractor is only able to bill for Chiropractic when an adjustment is performed.

One day, insurance companies will recognize the importance of proper neurological functioning and the maintenance thereof. Until then, your Upper Cervical Doctor's goal will be to provide you and your family with care that is safe and affordable, especially for those that are willing to invest in themselves.

"Do you offer any family programs?"

Absolutely! Just as the whole family typically does when going to their dentist because everyone's teeth are important, you are encouraged to bring your whole family in to have their spines evaluated because optimal well-being depends on a healthy spine and nerve system. When the family is under care together, not only is it more affordable, but a special healing bond is formed.

"How do I know if Upper Cervical Chiropractic is for me?"

Neurologic examinations and subsequent spinal imaging (via x-ray or CT) performed by Upper Cervical Chiropractors are designed to assess your candidacy for Upper Cervical Care. These tests answer the above question directly and conclusively.

The vertebral subluxation is very common on account of the frequency that traumas occur throughout life, particularly during the earlier years. Because it causes neurologic dysfunction, the Atlas (C1) or Axis (C2) misalignment immediately or eventually creates many obvious signs and symptoms in most people, who often then learn about Upper Cervical Chiropractic after running the gamut of various treatment-oriented options. That said, no matter if you are seeking causative answers to short or long-term health issues or you are just looking to maximize your potential – if you are seeking to have that "edge," to have clarity in your thinking, to be a better spouse or parent, or if you desire to be your best when it comes to being an athlete or student – then Upper Cervical Chiropractic is for you!

"WILL MASSAGE, PHYSICAL THERAPY, OR EXERCISE CAUSE MY SPINE TO GO OUT OF ADJUSTMENT?"

This question is quite difficult to answer because the different types of massage, physical therapy, or body work vary from one practitioner to another.

A massage therapist is trained to locate muscle imbalances, spasms, or trigger points ("knots") and then massage both muscles and other soft tissues with the intention of relieving pain, restoring structural/body balance, and aiding in recovery from soft tissue injuries. Keep in mind that the Atlas (C1) vertebra is supported and held in position by muscles rather than having a locking joint. So, if a massage therapist were to stretch, apply pressure to, or manipulate any of the muscles in the spine inappropriately, he/she could very well cause the spine to shift out of adjustment without either party being aware of it.

Not every massage will "throw off" your adjustment; typically your doctor will recommend that if you were to get one, it should be shoulders-down and the neck musculature should be left alone so as not to inadvertently interfere with your recovery (especially during the initial phase of Upper Cervical Care). Once you can hold the adjustment consistently and your spine stabilizes, your Upper Cervical Chiropractor will let you know that it is safe to reduce the restrictions on your massages.

Physical and Occupational therapists (PTs and OTs) are practitioners that help to rehabilitate injured people in order to recover their functional movement, manage their pain, and/or improve their activities of daily living. This is done with exercise, stretching, joint manipulation, or other modalities such as muscle stimulation (TENS), ultrasound, or laser therapy. As with massage, care should be taken not to disrupt the natural re-adaptation process facilitated by Upper Cervical Care.

Regardless of which therapy, care, or workout regimen one is currently utilizing, an optimally functioning nerve system will only add benefit to that therapy and speed up your recovery while under their guidance. Your therapist or trainer should be informed about the care you are receiving, as they should want to help protect your spine from losing its adjustment as well.

"DOES IT MATTER WHAT TYPE OF PILLOW OR MATTRESS I USE, AND WHAT SLEEP POSITION IS THE BEST FOR ME?"

Can you believe that a third of your life is spent sleeping? As crazy as that sounds, it is true. That means if you were to live to 90 years old, you would have slept for 30 years of your life! All the more reason why the type of mattress and pillow you use is imperative to supporting your spine properly when you sleep.

Your mattress should be on the relatively firmer side. A Sleep Number or Tempurpedic "memory foam" type of mattress will support the spine well, as they are designed to keep your body from "dipping" into the mattress like a hammock.

The most important aspect of sleeping, is to ensure that your neck is being correctly supported; the cervical "contour" pillows typically have two different sized "humps" (shaped like the curve that should be in your neck) to support your neck when laying on your back or your side.

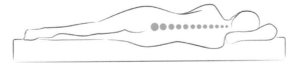

You should never sleep on your stomach. By doing so, the head is turned 90 degrees and the leg to the side of where the head is turned is elevated as well. The body then attempts to support the head by placing the arms underneath the pillow, causing both the spinal muscles and joints to be in a compromised position. To top it off, the vertebral arteries that travel up and through the vertebrae in your neck become kinked due to the 90 degree head angle, causing diminished blood and oxygen supply to the brain. Stomach sleepers often awake irritable and unrested with neck and back pain or stiffness.

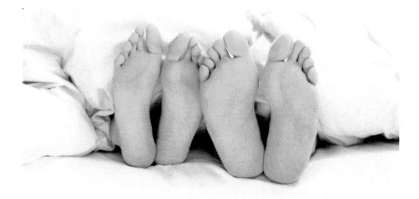

The ideal sleeping position is to be anatomically correct, which means sleeping on your back. If at all possible, start in that position for at least 10 minutes and then shift to your side. Resting your neck on the contour pillow will help relax the muscles and joints as your spine will be in a neutral (untwisted) position.

Frankly, since the goal is to hold your adjustment for a prolonged period of time, proper sleeping environment and habits are a must.

"What is the difference between an Upper Cervical Chiropractor and a regular Chiropractor?"

This question is a slippery slope because, unfortunately, the Chiropractic profession is a like box of chocolates – one never really knows what they are going to get when seeking a Chiropractor. Many Chiropractors offer acupuncture or physical therapy, or promote vitamins, shoe lifts, diets and weight loss, massage, stretches, and/or exercise. Chiropractors, generally, are among the few professionals that tend to be "jacks of all trades" rather than "staying in their own lane." On top of that, most Chiropractors believe that the more adjustments you get, the better off you are.

If you were to ask somebody what they do for living and they told you that they were an attorney, you would probably reply with, "What kind of law do you practice?" The same is actually true when speaking to a Chiropractor. There are hundreds of different types of Chiropractors and they all have their own spin and justification on why they do what they do.

Upper Cervical is a strict discipline of Chiropractic that is not only safe and gentle for anyone at any age, but it also applies scientific principles for knowing exactly how and when/when not to adjust those receiving this unique type of care. In the event that your Upper Cervical Chiropractor locates where the spine is compromised (structurally and neurologically), the particular upper cervical vertebra causing that compromise would require an adjustment, which would restore proper function to the body; otherwise, the body would be left alone to do what it is designed to do. No other profession can offer that to you.

"Is the Upper Cervical Chiropractic adjustment safe?"

One of the many unique adjusting attributes of an Upper Cervical Chiropractor is that they do not twist, pop, extend the head, or cause any type of muscle strain to the neck.

There has been controversy over the topic about Chiropractors causing injury or stroke. A stroke is when a small piece of plaque breaks free from the inner wall of an artery and travels up to the brain. There is also another condition called cervical artery dissection (tearing of the artery), which is due to the neck being over-rotated; this can cause a clot to form and possibly lead to a stroke. Both conditions can be due to gross rotational (twisting) type manipulations of the head and neck.

The Upper Cervical adjustment eliminates the above concerns because of the precise calculations made, along with the minimal amount of force it takes to shift the Atlas (or Axis) vertebra out of its abnormal position. The vertebral arteries within the spine, as well as other structures, are never compromised because both your head and spine are placed in a neutral position when receiving an adjustment. Hence, the Upper Cervical adjustment is safe for the entire family, regardless of age.

"Does the Upper Cervical adjustment hurt?"

The adjustment itself should never hurt, although it may feel a little sensitive or slightly uncomfortable in the beginning of care because your spine has been stuck in an abnormal position for several years to decades and your muscles and ligaments have adapted to the abnormal positioning. Those who have never received an Upper Cervical Chiropractic adjustment most likely have joints in their spines that have been remodelled, like a car tire having worn from improper wheel alignment. Unlocking that misaligned vertebra may cause tenderness due to muscle memory and significant changes in the tissues surrounding that vertebra.

However, the majority of those that receive an Upper Cervical Chiropractic adjustment have surprised looks on their faces immediately afterward, as if to say, "That's it?"

Sometimes in life, it is the simplest things that make the biggest difference.

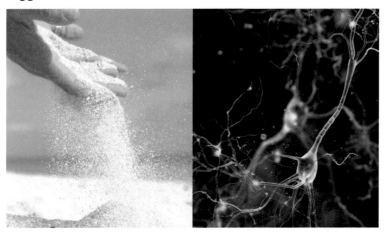

WHEN GRAINS OF SAND COME TOGETHER, IT FORMS A BEACH. WHEN TRILLIONS UPON TRILLIONS OF CELLS WORK TOGETHER, IT FORMS A BODY. IN LIFE, THE SMALLEST THINGS MAKE THE BIGGEST DIFFERENCE.

"WILL I HEAR OR FEEL ANYTHING DURING THE ADJUSTMENT?"

The experience can vary on account of which type of Upper Cervical Doctor you are seeing. Some doctors use instrumentation to make the spinal adjustment, others lay you on your side and use their hands, while some others place you into a kneeling position with your torso laying on the adjustment table. Depending on what type of application or procedure is utilized for your adjustment, you may hear a clicking type of noise or hear the adjustment table drop or shift.

When an Upper Cervical Chiropractic adjustment is made, people often feel an instantaneous blood flow change with a warm and tingling feeling in their head or neck regions; some notice that their sinuses clear immediately and others feel very relaxed; there are occasions when people get emotional and shed a few tears; some may feel slightly lightheaded due to the shift in their blood pressure; some may also notice a difference in their respiratory volumes, which means the lungs are better able to take in more air and that deeper breaths can be taken. All of these sensations are completely normal.

"WHAT WILL I FEEL AFTER MY ADJUSTMENT WHILE IN THE RESTING SUITE?"

During the resting period, you may experience a deeper, relaxed state as your body shifts into neurological balance or ease. Many fall asleep (which is ideal), as the mind becomes completely relaxed. Some get cold, while others get warm.

You may feel localized warm spots in joints, breathe much deeper, and feel a sense of mental calmness, as if the "fog has been lifted"; many people feel their bodies/spines shifting and sometimes hear a clicking or popping noise (pressure being released from joints that were stuck in compensation), while others feel twitches or muscles shifting; you may notice a subtle tingling sensation throughout your body, especially in your arms and legs; sinus drainage and many other constructive changes can also occur when your nerve system is restored back to proper functioning.

Keep in mind that no two people have the same reaction, because no two spines are neurologically or structurally compromised alike.

"IS IT POSSIBLE TO HAVE ADVERSE REACTIONS AFTER AN ADJUSTMENT?"

It is common for the body to have different types of soreness or stiffness during the restorative phase of care, but unlike an adverse reaction associated with a treatment-oriented approach (like pharmaceuticals), these responses are part of the healing process. There is a difference between feeling uncomfortable because your body is getting worse versus feeling uncomfortable because your body is trying to get better. Context is key. When an adjustment is made, the newly established position of the head and spine causes the neck muscles, ligaments, and joints to adapt to the structural

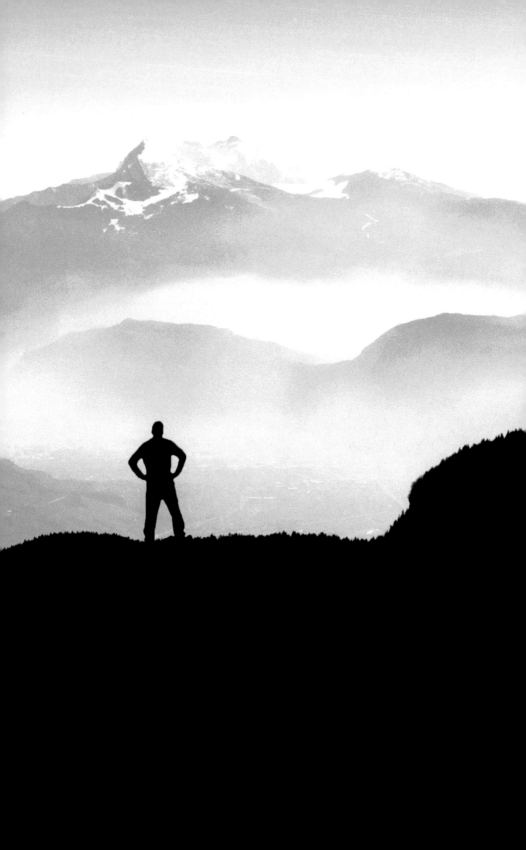

changes; abnormal has likely become normal for you, after all. If you experience old or new discomforts throughout your body, these are typically signs or symptoms that your body is in a state of rebalancing and repairing from past falls, accidents, or emotional traumas. The immediate rebalancing will usually last 2 to 3 weeks while chronic conditions may have a much longer healing time (see Chapter 10: Retracing to get a better understanding of the healing process)

"WHAT IS THE SUCCESS RATE OF UPPER CERVICAL CARE?"

Everyone's body is different. Just as people look different on the outside, people are different on the inside. The medical profession tends to treat people with the same diagnosis the same way, even though everyone is unique. Upper Cervical Chiropractors recognize that we are all different and therefore every person will have their own healing process or time frame.

When it comes to attaining some sort of result, most people see an immediate change within the first few weeks after their initial Upper Cervical adjustment. Depending on how long you have been experiencing your health issue, most long-term healing responses are gradual and can take several months or years depending on the severity of the condition.

Just as a mechanic tunes up a car that has had some "wear and tear," the Upper Cervical Chiropractor seeks to do the same for your body. By keeping your spine neurologically "tuned up," you give yourself the best chance at life. If you are just a few weeks old, a teenager, in your 40s, or ready to retire – regardless of age, health condition, or "wear and tear" you may have experienced – everyone benefits by having a properly functioning nerve system.

"What should I do over the next few days and weeks after my Upper Cervical adjustment?"

The goal is to have your spine hold the adjustment in place for a prolonged period of time. Everyone will hold their adjustment for a different time frame, as no two spines are neurologically or structurally alike. Some people will hold for several days, while others hold several weeks or months, eventually even years. The longer one is under care, the opportunity to hold the adjustment for an extended period of time is much greater due to having reestablished both normal function and a balanced spinal structure. This will not only stabilize the body physically, but the immune, respiratory, and cardiovascular systems will also be affected in a positive manner.

To help positively influence how long you can hold, please be "head and neck conscious" and refrain from putting any stress or strain on the head or neck region for the few weeks following an Upper Cervical adjustment. Some of those stressors include texting, sleeping on your stomach or not using a contour pillow, strenuous weight lifting or exercise habits, watching TV in bed with the head/neck propped up, and poor ergonomic posture while at work, just to name a few (see Chapter 9: Maintaining the Adjustment).

"Are there things that can inhibit my healing?"

The body and the mind are not big fans of stress, which can block or interfere with the body's natural healing process. Lifestyle habits like a poor diet and being sedentary, the use of medications, and believe it or not, a negative mindset are some of the many variables that can inhibit healing.

Medications (whether over-the-counter or prescribed) block the body's ability to restore itself back to normal; they are synthetic substances that either stimulate or inhibit the body's normal functioning, and they often slow down the body's ability to heal. When you are experiencing healing symptoms and the body is attempting to either rid itself of toxins or the spine is making structural changes, it may not be comfortable. Unfortunately, most people resort to medications to alleviate any of the discomfort when these healing symptoms are actually normal signs of restoration. That does not mean that you will not receive the benefits of Upper Cervical Care if you have poor lifestyle habits or are on medications, just that these things will alter your ability to achieve the maximum benefits regarding your health and well-being. Remember that your Upper Cervical Doctor did not prescribe or recommend any type of medications and it is NOT the role or the intent of your Upper Cervical Doctor to remove any medications; that is between you and the prescribing doctor.

The number one inhibitor of healing, is a negative mindset. Thoughts always become things, hence the importance of having a positive attitude geared towards the life that you desire. When in agreement with your Upper Cervical Doctor's intention and recommendations, only good things can come of it. In contrast, when you constantly doubt the care that your doctor is providing or you are unwilling to make any changes to your lifestyle, you will not only waste your time and money, but you will begin to blame others for your inability to heal. "What the mind believes, the body achieves."

"WHEN IS A GOOD AGE TO START HAVING MY SPINE CHECKED?"

Shortly after birth, ideally.

The birthing process for both the mother and newborn can be very traumatic. Most pregnant women today are told by their doctor how, when, and where the birth is going to take place. Unfortunately, in today's "go-go-go" world, the birth is scheduled to accommodate the doctor's schedule. This often leads to the use of unnecessary chemicals for both managing pain and speeding up the birthing process by inducement. No other species interferes with this process.

Once the mother is given medications, the nerve system responds by causing uterine contractions to expedite the delivery. All too often the mother is then given an epidural to prevent any possible discomfort, along with pitocin, the synthetic version of oxytocin, a natural hormone all females produce that helps the uterus contract during labor.

The body then experiences medication-induced contractions that force the fetus's head towards the not yet fully dilated cervix. This triggers a severe pain response, prompting the epidural; that is if the mother has not already been given an epidural for the discomfort, seeing as most women today have been made so afraid of giving birth that the epidural is often given before the birth process even begins! The epidural numbs the nerves within the spine, similar to novocain for a tooth, but when the mother is told to push, she cannot feel what she is pushing, thus putting undue pressure onto the head and neck of her newborn. To add "fuel to the fire," the involuntary, forced contractions from pitocin add to the pain and possible head and neck trauma.

Once the fetus is through the cervix and the head begins to "crown" (reveal itself), the mother continues to push while laying propped up on her back with her legs elevated, causing a narrower vaginal opening, and almost 100% of the time, the practitioner that is facilitating the birth then uses his/her fingers to get a hold of the head. Once the fingers are around the head, the delivery is then assisted by pulling the head to fully extract the fetus. At least 75% of the time, this unnecessarily strenuous process causes muscle, ligament, head, and neck injury. The same scenario, if not worse, occurs when a caesarian (C) section is performed. Unfortunately, this has become the norm, thus creating a sub-par environment for the newborn to have its first experience of life; most babies are subluxated during birth.

This is why your Upper Cervical Chiropractor would tell you that the best age to start care is the moment you are born. It is safe, gentle, and benefits the entire family regardless of age.

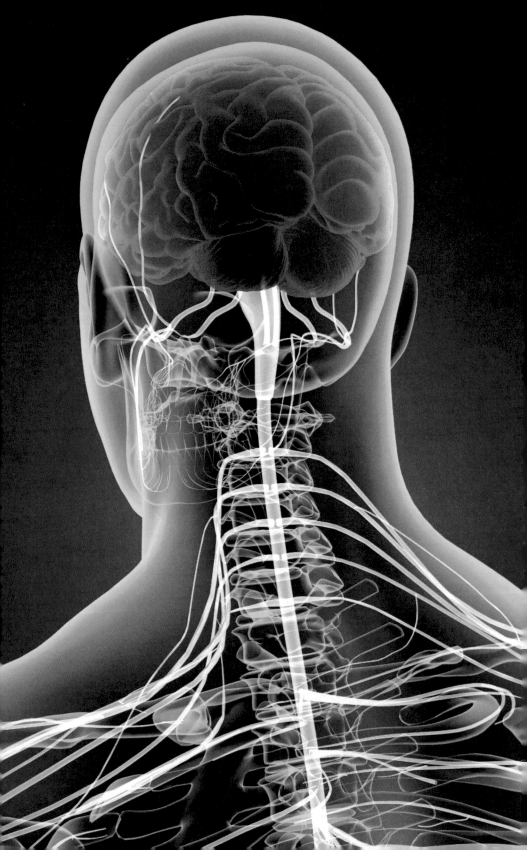

"How often should I be adjusted?"

Remember that the goal of your Upper Cervical Doctor is to only adjust your spine when necessary. This is what makes Upper Cervical Care different and unique compared to other types of Chiropractic within the profession. Many Chiropractors initially adjust people 2 to 3 times per week for several weeks or months. Upper Cervical Chiropractic offices do not operate like that at all. Typically, your Upper Cervical Doctor will want to see you once a week (maybe twice a week depending on the severity of the case) for the first month or so. Then, they begin to taper your visits down depending on how well your spine is holding the adjustment. The longer your spine remains in a neurologically stable state, the quicker one has the potential to heal.

Your body does not need any assistance beyond the removal of interference to its functioning. You WILL NOT have to be adjusted on every visit. Honestly, most people, after about 4 to 6 months of care, will begin to hold their adjustment for a month or two at a time, hence why you would only need to be seen once a month thereafter. Think of it like taking care of a plant. How often should you water a plant? You should water the plant only when it needs it. With that same understanding, your spine should be adjusted only when it needs it as well.

"How long will I need to be under care?"

That is completely up to you. When people invest their time and money by joining a gym, eating organic foods, and choosing Upper Cervical Chiropractic Care as part of their lifestyles, only good can come of it. Your body is the only place that YOU are going to live, so why not do your best to take care of it? Think of it like getting braces. Why invest the money to straighten your teeth if you are unwilling to later wear the retainer to keep them straight?

Your body has been made to take care of itself; give your body what it needs and let it do what it was designed to do. The transformation that your body undergoes during the first 12 months of care is unlike anything you will ever experience. Once the body is in a stable neurological and structural position, then maintaining it is relatively simple, especially if one begins care at an early age.

So, how long should one be under Upper Cervical Care? No two people would answer that question the same. However, if you were to ask Upper Cervical Doctors how long they plan on having their spines checked, they would tell you "for the rest of our lives." If diet, exercise, and rest make sense, then why not incorporate proper nerve system functioning to your lifestyle as well? Being the best version of you emotionally and physically – having that "edge" in life – all starts with a properly functioning nerve system.

"WHAT ABOUT THE REST OF MY SPINE?"

In the beginning of this book, we introduced the Upper Cervical Chiropractic concept illustrating how 22 of the 24 vertebrae within your spine possess an interlocking joint, thus restricting motion to protect the nerves.

The infrared spinal scan that is utilized to identify if your spine has any neurological compromise can and should be applied to the entire spine after your initial Upper Cervical spinal adjustment to ensure that your neurologic dysfunction has been restored both at the base of your skull as well as the remainder of the spine. Just about every nerve in your spine originates within the Atlas vertebra, and when it subluxates (see Chapter 3), your entire spine structurally and neurologically begins to compensate as well. Therefore, once the neurological compromise is restored, the entire spine will adapt and adjust accordingly.

"Upper Cervical Chiropractors are full spine practitioners, they simply apply the full spine adjustment via the upper cervical spine."

"DOES MY TMJ HAVE ANYTHING TO DO WITH MY SPINE?"

TMJ function is dependent upon the teeth fitting together properly as well as proper upper cervical spinal mechanics.

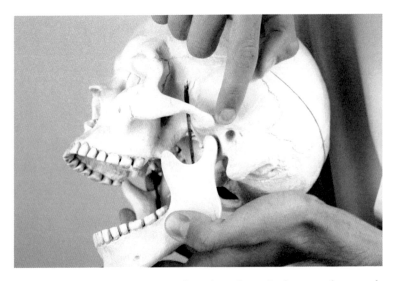

If either your teeth or your head and neck do not align with one another, your TMJ (temporomandibular joint) will be displaced. Many studies, websites, and books link dysfunction of the TMJ or cranial-cervical-mandibular disorders to multiple symptoms, including but not limited to Meniere's disease, decreased hearing, fullness in the ears, headaches, dizziness, vertigo, nausea, difficulty balancing, difficulty swallowing, neck and shoulder soreness, clicking and grinding sounds in the jaw joints, limited mouth opening/movement, visual disturbances, and in some cases neurological conditions like trigeminal neuralgia.

The muscles in the face, head, and neck all work together to help maintain your skull on top of the spine with the task of attaining the most optimal, properly balanced position.

Your mandible (jaw) is what controls the bottom teeth; your top teeth, meanwhile, are attached to what is called the maxilla, which is also part of your skull. So the big question is, "What is controlling your skull's position?" If you guessed your Atlas, then you would be right. Your skull rests on top of the Atlas, and when the Atlas misaligns (subluxates), then the head shifts to one side causing the spine, joints, and muscles to accommodate to the abnormal position. This is how the TMJ becomes misaligned as well. Many dentists, oral surgeons, and orthodontists attempt to lineup the jaw (mandible) while the head is out of balance, which makes their jobs very challenging. When your Atlas is adjusted, both the head and spine align, as well as the TMJ.

"CAN YOU ADJUST SOMEONE THAT IS PREGNANT?"

If a woman was to become pregnant, her own nerve supply becomes responsible for not one, but two different bodies, as she is the host for the fetus. Over the next 9 months, her body will completely transform structurally, physiologically, and emotionally. So, it is imperative that the mother's body be neurologically and structurally sound. When pregnant, the pelvis and spine are in a new position due to the growth of the fetus, so when the spine is in alignment, the pelvis is then in an ideal position for delivery. Once the baby is born, having his/her spine checked will ensure that your child starts off on the right foot when it comes to sleeping habits, demeanor, a strong immune system, and overall health.

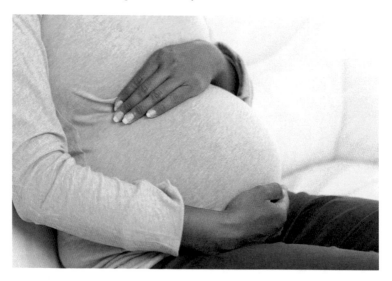

"CAN I STILL BE ADJUSTED IF I HAVE HAD SPINAL SURGERY?"

Unfortunately, when most hear the word "Chiropractic," they think about someone that twists and pops your back. Upper Cervical Chiropractors are adamant that there be no type of twisting or popping of the spine. Simply speaking, Upper

Cervical Care aims to ensure that the head is sitting properly on top of the spine for optimal neurological communication from the brain to the body. Spinal surgery is rarely ever performed at the upper most portion of the spine, but rather below this area due to either spinal degeneration, trauma, and/or improper lifting. It is quite safe for those who have had spinal surgery to be under this type of care.

"DO ALL CHIROPRACTORS ADJUST THE UPPER CERVICAL PART OF THE SPINE?"

Just about every Chiropractor has the intention to adjust the upper cervical spine, but very few are trained to do it correctly. In order to adjust the Atlas or Axis from its abnormal position, a gentle and precise force is required without any twisting of the head or neck because of the relational shape of the joints that the skull and the Atlas possess; the Atlas has two cup-like joints that your skull rests upon, similar to holding a bowling ball with both hands supporting it from underneath. If you were to turn your head, it would rotate / spin on those two joints. It therefore takes a very specific correction to adjust the Atlas or Axis properly.

Any twisting of the spine will cause the joints below the Atlas to "lock out," and if the force is great enough, it will cause them to make a popping sound (called a cavitation) similar to cracking your knuckles. The popping is nitrogen gas leaving the joint capsule (a balloon like structure that holds the joint together), NOT an adjustment. Unfortunately, the majority of the Chiropractic profession has very little knowledge of how to apply an Upper Cervical Chiropractic adjustment.

"MY PRIMARY PHYSICIAN THINKS YOU ARE NOT A REAL DOCTOR."

According to Webster's dictionary, doctor means teacher or educator. A "real doctor" could be a psychologist, veterinarian, dentist, pastor, lawyer, surgeon, or musician; the list goes on and on. Each one has earned the highest scholastic ranking regarding their trade.

A medical doctor is one that aims to treat a disease or condition with the use of medications and/or surgery.

The Doctor of Chiropractic is one that focuses on spinal function to ensure that the body is both neurologically and structurally sound. They are both unique to their field and expertise and offer two completely different types of care, similar to the difference between a carpenter and a plumber. In a scholastic comparison, Chiropractors have roughly 300 more class hours compared to your primary medical doctor.

Any time a doctor, practitioner, or professional seeks to sway a patient or client's decision based on their own beliefs or opinions, it speaks volumes about their knowledge on the subject, and contradicts what should be the primary goal: to help you to become a better you within their own field of expertise.

"MY D.O. (DOCTOR OF OSTEOPATHY) AND PT (PHYSICAL THERAPIST) SAID THEY CAN ADJUST THE SPINE TOO."

Per Google...The D.O. and PT both perform manipulations to the spine and extremities to treat muscle pain and dysfunctions related to the entire skeletal system, but neither perform adjustments. The Chiropractic adjustment is intended to restore the body to good working order, to help it regulate itself, and to bring it to a proper state or position. A Chiropractor (D.C.) is trained to "adjust" both the spine and extremities.

As much as it is a play on words, the definitions are quite vague, mostly to avoid conflict between the professions. It is a political thing and it does not explain how each of the practitioners can uniquely help the body to function properly. If a D.O. or PT states that they are "adjusting" the spine similarly to the Chiropractor, the same question should be asked to the D.O or PT; "Can a Chiropractor manipulate like a D.O. or PT?"

An adjustment can only take place within the spine. In order for the spine to be subluxated, it must have a joint misalignment, narrowing of the opening through which a nerve exits, and it must cause neurological dysfunction to that nerve. Without a vertebra in the spine possessing those

3 qualifications, the attempt to perform an adjustment would be impossible.

The D.O., PT, and general D.C. have similar intentions to improve the body's ability to function. They each have their own understanding and intention, but lack the scientific proof that their manipulation or adjustment occurred. Hearing a "popping" sound does not prove that a manipulation or adjustment occurred. Neither the D.O. or PT (or most Chiropractors) have a way of knowing if what they did was constructive to either the extremity or spine because no type of "before and after" objective gauge is typically ever utilized. Please understand that in no way is this a mockery of any sort, as this type of debate has been going on for over a century.

However, your Upper Cervical Doctor uses imaging (X-Rays, MRI, or CT) to reveal the structural state of the spine and infrared thermography to identify any neurological compromise(s). Moreover, the infrared thermography is utilized before and after the spinal adjustment to prove that nerve function was properly restored, unlike the D.O. or PT.

Respectfully, until the D.O. or PT utilizes some sort of objective gauge to prove their work, they have no way of knowing if "they can adjust the spine too."

"I DON'T FEEL WELL AND YOU ARE NOT GOING TO ADJUST ME? WHY NOT?"

The nurse or medical doctor typically asks, "What brings you in today?" That is because most go to see the medical doctor when experiencing some sort of pain or symptom. Their protocol is to ask several questions regarding your symptoms and then perform several different exams in the attempt to identify what body part is malfunctioning. Then, the treatment is to give you a drug designed to speed up or slow down the nerve supply in hopes of restoring the body back to health. If you are having diarrhea, for instance, a drug is given to slow down the colon; conversely, if you have constipation, a drug is given to speed it up. Regardless of the type of medication, pharmaceuticals are NOT designed to allow your nerve supply to function the way it was intended: free of any compromise.

Although sympathetic to your discomfort, the job of the Upper Cervical Chiropractor is to gauge how well the nerve system is functioning. The Upper Cervical Doctor will certainly not disregard how you are feeling, but your symptoms do not dictate how, when, or where to provide care. Symptoms are not necessarily an indication that your body is not functioning properly, especially during the initial phase of care (see Chapter 10: Retracing). The majority of the time, symptoms are part of the healing process. When a neurological spinal scan is performed, often your spine will be "clear" of any neurological compromise (see Chapter 9: Maintaining the Adjustment), although you may not be feeling well at that particular point in time. Remember, the premise behind this type of care is to ensure that your spine is free of any neurological compromise. The body does not need any assistance, just no interference to its functioning (see Chapter 8: The 3-Ts).

"When can I stop taking my medication?"

Medications are not part of Chiropractic; they never were and hopefully they never will be because they completely go against the philosophy and principles of Chiropractic. Medicine's premise is that sickness can only be restored from an outside source (medications or surgery), while Chiropractors believe that if the problem comes from the inside, then the solution to that problem does too.

When a Chiropractor aims to assist someone getting off of their medications, it is not Chiropractic, nor is it legal. "Do people get off of their prescriptions while under care?" Absolutely! When function is restored to the nerve system, malfunctioning parts of the body are given the ability to heal themselves; when the nerve system is monitored over an extended period of time, symptoms and lab data reveal that healing and restoration occurred. It is at this point that people seek to get off of their medications. If you are interested in getting off of your medications, that decision is between you and the prescribing doctor.

"If I had a problem with my brainstem or spinal cord, wouldn't I know it?"

Believe it or not, the weight of a dime on a spinal nerve will alter the nerve function up to 60%, and yet you would never know it. The nerves that exit the spine possess what are called "proprioceptors", "nociceptors" and "mechanoreceptors". These sensory nerve receptors are responsible for position, movement, and pain. When your spine is subluxated (Atlas or Axis misalignment), it causes a neurological disturbance affecting the entire spinal column. Yet, it is impossible to feel it because the brain and spinal cord lack any pain or sensory nerve fibers; if they did, pain would be debilitating. Such is why having your spine checked at least once a month to ensure neurological integrity is so important.

"I feel fine, why would I still need care?"

If your dentist recommends that you have your teeth checked every 6 months or a mechanic recommends that you have your oil changed every 3,000 to 5,000 miles, would you just wait until you had pain in your mouth from a degenerated tooth or wait until the check engine light comes on in your car? Your spine is far more dynamic than your teeth or your automobile.

Having your spine examined (once a month) to ensure that your nerve system is functioning properly just makes sense. When it comes to health, most have been taught that if you do not have any type of pain or symptom, then the body must be healthy, but health is not that black and white. Health should never be gauged on how well you are feeling, but rather on how well the body is functioning.

CHAPTER 12:

YOU'VE GOT SOME NERVE!

Your Upper Cervical Doctor is board certified and thoroughly trained to detect both the abnormal structural issues and neurological dysfunction of the spine. The question often arises as to why the Chiropractor cannot fix the spine and restore nerve function immediately. Rest assured, when your doctor reviews the data collected from your day one examinations, you will have a better grasp of your spine and neurological issues and how they are related to your condition.

When the specific, tailor-made adjustment is administered to your subluxated spine, the vertebra is then returned to its normal position; and when this occurs, the muscles and ligaments must then adapt to the new positioning of your spine, creating an opportunity for your spine to "hold" the Atlas vertebra properly. Due to daily stressors – thoughts, traumas, and toxins (see Chapter 8: The 3-Ts) – the odds of your spine returning back to its previous abnormal positioning are probable. Thus, periodic (monthly) spinal and neurological exams are imperative to give your body the best opportunity to maintain its optimal function.

An Upper Cervical Chiropractor often hears:

- "My doctor said there's nothing more he/she can do."
- "I take medications for migraines and they have not gone away."
- "You can't help me, I have cancer."
- "I will be on medication for the rest of my life."
- "I have had surgery; it's too late."
- "Diabetes runs in the family, I'll probably get it."
- "I have neuropathy, so what's the point?"
- "I have high blood pressure, reflux, and high cholesterol. I can't be fixed; I have too many things that are going wrong."
- "My child is on their third round of antibiotics for ear infections."

The human list of complaints, worries, skepticism, and doubts never ends. Keep in mind that if your problem came from the inside, so must the answer to that problem. Every cell, tissue, and organ is connected to your nerve system. Our creator put logic in the nerve; it is called the NEURO-LOGIC system after all. Therefore, the proper functioning of your nerve system is imperative to your overall health and well-being.

Hopefully by now you get the gist that Upper Cervical Chiropractic is not about fixing any type of condition, treating any particular issue, or getting you out of pain. It is about giving your body and your mind the ability to thrive both physically and emotionally on every level regardless of age, race, or the condition of your health.

Simply speaking, everyone deserves the opportunity to experience life to its fullest. To us, It Just Makes Sense.

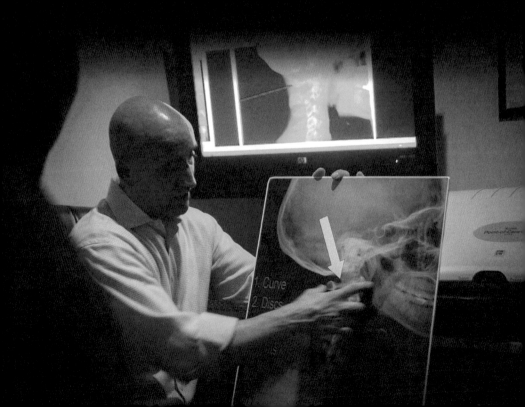

PEOPLE SAY,
"WE ONLY LIVE ONCE."
WE RESPECTFULLY DISAGREE.

YOU ONLY DIE ONCE, BUT YOU GET A CHANCE
TO LIVE EVERY DAY. THE UPPER CERVICAL
CHIROPRACTIC VISION AND MISSION IS TO GIVE
YOU AND YOUR FAMILY THE OPPORTUNITY TO
EXPERIENCE A BETTER QUALITY OF LIFE.

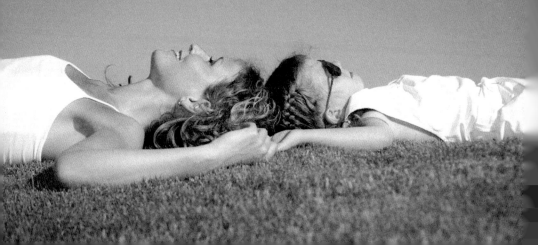

Acknowledgements

To those special few that blessed me with their wisdom, gifts, talents, and skills who planted a seed that would eventually germinate into me becoming the ChiropracTOR that I am today, know that I am eternally grateful.

- **Dr. Flavian Santavicca** for introducing me to Chiropractic

- **Dr. Robert Kessinger** for sharing his heart and years of ChiropracTIC mentoring

- **Dr. Michael Kale** for his passion and teachings

- **Dr. John Strazewski** for his HIO / toggle recoil wisdom

- **Dr. John Goodfellow** for his passion and straight principles

Thank you to those that went above and beyond that helped make this book happen…

- **Megan O'Brien** for putting up with my many requests regarding editing and changes as she was the wonderful soul that designed the book.

- **Dr. Daniel Walthers** for the use of the many beautiful Chiropractic illustrations.

- **Dr. Chad McIntyre** for your incredible writing, passion, and editing abilities.

Thank you to all of the Upper Cervical Chiropractors that have chosen to "stay the course" and to all of the "Straights" that went to jail for a cause bigger than themselves. Thank you Dr. B.J. Palmer for standing up for what you knew was right. Know that your tireless work, heart, passion, wisdom, and dedication to and for the profession will forever be revered as it is my aim to protect the sacred trust.

To those that allowed me to be part of their lives as they have been a huge part of mine… I thank you! To my parents who never stopped me from being me. To my wife who puts up with the "go-go-go Eddie Energy" and lets me be as a husband, father, and doctor.

To Sue Wear for supporting and helping me serve the subluxated while writing this book. To Micheal Gebben for your never-ending passion that keeps me keeping on. To the 10,000+ people that have been under my care over the past 20 years and to the 200+ students and doctors that I have personally been able to either "take under my wing" and/or mentor. Oh, and I cannot forget the naysayers, thank you for fueling my why.

Most importantly, I thank God for the divine above-down, inside-out blessing that flows into my head, through my heart, and is delivered via my hands called the Adjustment with that "Extra-Something."

I pray that the content in this book gives you hope and a new outlook on life as it did for me.

Forever Serving,

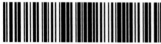

Made in the USA
Lexington, KY
11 September 2019